COSMETIC LASER THERAPY FOR BEGINNERS

Comprehensive Guide To Safe And Effective Treatments For Skin Rejuvenation, Wrinkle Reduction, Hair Removal, And Acne Scarring

DR SAWYER DIEGO

DISCLAMER

Nothing in this book should be interpreted as medical advice; it is meant exclusively for educational reasons. Regarding their specific health issues and treatment options, readers are urged to speak with licensed healthcare professionals. The publisher and author disclaim all liability for any errors or omissions in the material provided, as well as for any negative effects that may arise from using or abusing the information. Although every attempt has been taken to guarantee that the material in this book is correct as of the date of publishing, new research may have superseded some of the content because medical knowledge is always changing. It is recommended that readers confirm the most recent medical recommendations and guidelines. The reader of this book undertakes to release the author and publisher from any claims or liabilities resulting from the use of this information, and understands and accepts the inherent risks connected with healthcare decisions.

TABLE OF CONTENTS

CHAPTER ONE 11

  COSMETIC LASER THERAPY OVERVIEW..11

    KNOWING THE FUNDAMENTALS OF COSMETIC LASER THERAPY......11

    THE VALUE OF PROFESSIONAL ADVICE AND SAFETY 12

    EXAMINING VARIOUS COSMETIC LASER TREATMENT 13

    ADVANTAGES AND DRAWBACKS OF COSMETIC LASER 14

    WHAT THIS BEGINNER'S GUIDE WILL TEACH YOU 15

CHAPTER TWO 17

  SYNOPSIS OF COSMETIC LASER TREATMENT 17

    OVERVIEW OF LASER COSMETIC PROCEDURES 17

    THE DEVELOPMENT AND HISTORY OF LASER THERAPY....................18

    SKIN CONDITIONS THAT LASERS CAN TREAT 20

    HOW SKINCARE LASERS OPERATE...21

    SAFETY OBSERVATIONS AND SAFETY MEASURES 23

CHAPTER THREE 25

  COSMETIC LASER TREATMENT TYPES 25

    LASER ACNE AND ACNE SCAR TREATMENTS.................................25

    TECHNIQUES FOR LASER HAIR REMOVAL 26

    AGE-REDUCING LASER PROCEDURES...28

    PROCEDURES FOR LASER TATTOO REMOVAL 29

    TREATMENTS FOR VASCULAR LESIONS AND PIGMENTATION 31

CHAPTER FOUR 33

  SELECTING THE APPROPRIATE LASER THERAPY 33

    KNOWING YOUR SKIN TYPE AND IF IT'S GOOD FOR LASERS.............33

PROCESS OF CONSULTATION WITH A CLINICIAN OR 35

FACTORS AFFECTING THE EFFECTIVENESS OF TREATMENT..............36

TAILORING INTERVENTIONS TO INDIVIDUAL REQUIREMENTS 37

CONTROLLING RESULTS AND EXPECTATIONS 39

CHAPTER FIVE...41

GETTING READY FOR A LASER PROCEDURE 41

SKINCARE ROUTINE BEFORE TREATMENT 41

KEEPING OUT OF THE SUN AND TAKING OTHER PRECAUTIONS........42

POSSIBLE ADVERSE REACTIONS AND THEIR HANDLING 43

MENTAL READINESS FOR THE INTERVENTION PROCEDURE 45

THINGS TO PACK AND KNOW BEFORE TREATMENT DAY 46

CHAPTER SIX...49

COURSE OF THE LASER TREATMENT 49

DETAILED PROCESS OF AN ORDINARY LASER SESSION 49

FEELINGS OF UNCOMFORT DURING MEDICAL INTERVENTION 50

SAFETY PROCEDURES THAT PRACTITIONERS ADHERE TO..................51

EFFECTS AND CHANGES SEEN IN REAL-TIME 52

SPEAKING WITH YOUR PHYSICIAN THROUGHOUT THE 54

CHAPTER SEVEN 55

RECUPERATION AND AFTERCARE 55

AFTER-TREATMENT SKINCARE SCHEDULE 55

HANDLING TRANSIENT SIDE EFFECTS LIKE SWELLING OR..................56

REFRAINING FROM ACTIVITIES THAT MAY AFFECT REHAB................58

APPOINTMENTS FOR FOLLOW-UP AND THEIR SIGNIFICANCE 59

TIPS FOR LONG-TERM SKINCARE MAINTENANCE 61

CHAPTER EIGHT...63

TYPICAL LASER THERAPY CONCERNS 63

LASER TREATMENT SAFETY FOR VARIOUS SKIN TONES.....................63

THE DANGERS OF LASER THERAPY AND HOW TO REDUCE................64

EVALUATING LASER THERAPY IN COMPARISON TO OTHER..............66

DISPELLING MYTHS AND FALSE BELIEFS REGARDING LASER 67

COMPREHENDING INSURANCE COVERAGE AND FINANCIAL............69

CHAPTER NINE 71

FREQUENTLY ASKED QUESTIONS ON COSMETIC LASER TREATMENT ...71

HOW MANY APPOINTMENTS ARE USUALLY REQUIRED?...................71

IS IT POSSIBLE TO COMBINE LASER TREATMENTS WITH 72

HOW IS PAIN HANDLED DURING LASER THERAPY? IS LASER.............74

WHAT DISTINGUISHES THE DIFFERENT LASER TECHNOLOGIES? 75

HOW MUCH TIME DO LASER TREATMENT RESULTS LAST? 77

CHAPTER TEN 79

FUTURE DIRECTIONS FOR COSMETIC LASER TREATMENT 79

ADVANCEMENTS IN LASER TECHNOLOGY AND THERAPY METHODS 79

NEW DEVELOPMENTS IN NON-INVASIVE COSMETIC........................80

COMBINING ROBOTICS AND AI FOR LASER TREATMENTS.................82

USING DIGITAL TOOLS TO EMPOWER AND EDUCATE PATIENTS 83

ETHICS AND ENVIRONMENTAL ASPECTS OF LASER THERAPY............84

ABOUT THE BOOK

In this book, readers will delve into the foundational aspects of cosmetic laser therapy, starting with an exploration of its basics and the critical importance of safety under professional guidance. Understanding the nuances of different types of cosmetic laser treatments is crucial, from combating signs of aging with specialized treatments to achieving smooth skin through laser hair removal. The book not only covers the benefits these therapies offer but also addresses their limitations, ensuring a balanced perspective for prospective patients. "Cosmic Laser Therapy for Beginners" serves as a comprehensive introduction to the world of cosmetic laser treatments, providing essential knowledge and practical guidance for those new to this rapidly evolving field.

Preparing readers for what to anticipate from laser therapy is a crucial aspect of this guide. From comprehending the workings of laser technology to handling expectations and outcomes, each section is painstakingly written to equip readers with the knowledge necessary to make educated decisions. The significance of one-on-one consultations and the variables affecting treatment efficacy are emphasized, underscoring the necessity of individualized care catered to specific skin types and concerns.

Additionally, the book covers common concerns and misconceptions surrounding laser therapy, providing clarity on safety considerations, treatment durations, and financial implications. Finally, it thoroughly covers pre-treatment preparations and post-treatment care, guaranteeing readers are well-equipped with useful tips to enhance treatment outcomes and manage potential side effects effectively.

Future trends in cosmetic laser therapy are covered in detail in the book, along with technological developments like robotics and AI integration that highlight how non-invasive cosmetic procedures are changing. Ethical and environmental issues are also covered, highlighting the treatments' wider effects on patient-centered care and sustainability.

"Cosmetic Laser Therapy for Beginners" is an invaluable resource for anyone considering or curious about the transformative possibilities of cosmetic laser therapy. Its overall goal is to educate and empower readers with thorough insights into the world of laser skincare, ensuring they embark on their treatment journeys well-informed and confident in their choices.

CHAPTER ONE

COSMETIC LASER THERAPY OVERVIEW

KNOWING THE FUNDAMENTALS OF COSMETIC LASER THERAPY

Cosmetic laser therapy is a non-invasive light-based procedure that targets specific areas of concern, like wrinkles, scars, or pigmentation. The light is absorbed by the skin at specific wavelengths, and this absorption turns it into heat energy that stimulates the production of collagen and elastin fibers in the skin's deeper layers, helping to tighten and rejuvenate the skin over time, giving it a smoother, more youthful appearance.

Following each session, the patient may experience temporary redness or mild swelling, which usually goes away within a few hours to a few days. The procedure starts with a consultation during which the dermatologist or trained technician evaluates the patient's skin condition and discusses treatment goals. During the session, the patient may feel a slight warmth or tingling as the laser pulses are applied to the targeted areas. Multiple sessions may be necessary for optimal results depending on the treatment area and desired outcomes.

Though results may vary depending on individual skin types and conditions, a customized treatment plan is essential for achieving desired outcomes, cosmetic laser therapy is known for its versatility as it can address a wide range of skin concerns, including fine lines, wrinkles, acne scars, sunspots, and vascular lesions. Overall, cosmetic laser therapy offers a promising option for those looking to enhance their skin's appearance without undergoing invasive surgery.

THE VALUE OF PROFESSIONAL ADVICE AND SAFETY

Cosmetic laser therapy places a strong emphasis on safety, underscoring the importance of having qualified professionals trained in laser technology perform the procedure with precision and adherence to safety protocols, minimizing risks and maximizing effectiveness. These professionals assess each patient's skin type, medical history, and treatment goals to determine the most appropriate laser type and settings, providing individualized care.

It is recommended that patients disclose any medications, allergies, or previous skin treatments to their provider to minimize the possibility of adverse reactions. Patients who prioritize safety and seek treatment from licensed professionals can pursue cosmetic laser therapy with confidence, knowing they are in capable hands.

EXAMINING VARIOUS COSMETIC LASER TREATMENT OPTIONS

A few common types of cosmetic laser treatments are fractional lasers, which create microscopic treatment zones to stimulate collagen production, promoting skin rejuvenation with minimal downtime; ablative lasers, which remove thin layers of skin to treat wrinkles and scars; and non-ablative lasers, which penetrate deeper layers without damaging the skin's surface.

Apart from that, pigmented lesions like freckles and age spots, vascular conditions like rosacea and spider veins, and unwanted hair growth through laser hair removal procedures can all be targeted by laser treatments. Different wavelengths and techniques are employed for different outcomes in each type of laser treatment, demonstrating the versatility of cosmetic laser therapy in aesthetic enhancement.

ADVANTAGES AND DRAWBACKS OF COSMETIC LASER TREATMENT

Cosmetic laser therapy offers a variety of advantages, including better skin tone, texture, and overall appearance; by promoting the production of collagen, lasers can tighten loose skin, minimize wrinkles, and make scars and stretch marks less noticeable. Compared to surgical procedures, laser treatments are frequently less invasive, cause less discomfort, and require shorter recovery times, which appeals to those looking for non-surgical cosmetic improvements.

A thorough consultation is necessary to assess candidacy and manage expectations. While lasers are generally safe when used by trained professionals, there is a risk of temporary side effects such as redness, swelling, or changes in pigmentation. Additionally, certain skin types or medical conditions may not be suitable for laser treatments. Finally, results may vary depending on individual skin characteristics and treatment goals, requiring multiple sessions for optimal outcomes.

WHAT THIS BEGINNER'S GUIDE WILL TEACH YOU

With the help of this beginner's guide, readers will gain a thorough understanding of cosmetic laser therapy, from its basic principles to practical considerations and expected outcomes. They will also gain insight into the safety protocols and individualized care involved in laser treatments, as well as an expanded understanding of the diverse applications and targeted benefits that each type of cosmetic laser therapy offers.

In addition, the guide provides readers with the necessary information to make well-informed decisions regarding the pursuit of aesthetic enhancements by outlining the possible advantages and drawbacks of cosmetic laser therapy. It also sets reasonable expectations and highlights the significance of customized treatment plans, giving novices the tools they need to successfully navigate their journey towards healthier, more radiant skin through cosmetic laser therapy.

CHAPTER TWO

SYNOPSIS OF COSMETIC LASER TREATMENT

OVERVIEW OF LASER COSMETIC PROCEDURES

In contrast to invasive procedures, cosmetic laser treatments are non-surgical and usually involve minimal downtime, making them popular choices for people seeking noticeable improvements with fewer risks. Whether targeting wrinkles, scars, pigmentation issues, or unwanted hair, these treatments use focused laser light to stimulate collagen production, renew skin cells, and achieve smoother, more youthful skin.

Knowing how various types of lasers interact with the skin's layers to address particular concerns is essential to understanding the fundamentals of cosmetic laser treatments. Lasers can target underlying tissues without damaging the outer layers of the skin by penetrating the skin to precise depths with controlled beams of light, allowing for customized treatment plans that are tailored to individual skin types and conditions, ensuring optimal results with minimal discomfort.

During an initial consultation, practitioners evaluate skin concerns, go over treatment options, and explain expected outcomes and potential risks. Having a basic understanding of these concepts helps patients make educated decisions about their skincare journey, ensuring they receive individualized care that is in line with their aesthetic goals. Selecting a reputable clinic and skilled practitioner is essential for safe and effective laser treatments.

THE DEVELOPMENT AND HISTORY OF LASER THERAPY

The first laser was created in the 1960s, which was a significant advancement in the medical and cosmetic sciences. Lasers were initially used for scientific research, but they soon found use in a variety of fields, including aesthetic medicine and dermatology.

As technology has advanced over the years, laser devices have become more precise, safe, and effective in treating a wide range of skin conditions.

Today, laser therapy is widely recognized for its ability to rejuvenate skin, reduce signs of aging, and enhance overall skin health. The evolution of laser therapy in skincare is a reflection of ongoing research and innovation, leading to the development of different laser types tailored to specific skin concerns. These advancements have broadened treatment options and improved patient outcomes. Examples of these include ablative lasers, which vaporize skin tissue, and non-ablative lasers, which target underlying layers without damaging the surface.

Understanding this evolution highlights the significance of seeking treatments from qualified professionals in accredited facilities to maximize safety and efficacy. Modern lasers incorporate sophisticated cooling systems and wavelength adjustments to minimize discomfort and reduce the risk of adverse effects.

Clinicians undergo specialized training to operate these devices safely; ensuring patients receive optimal care and achieve desired cosmetic outcomes.

SKIN CONDITIONS THAT LASERS CAN TREAT

Cosmetic lasers are highly adaptable and can be used to treat a wide range of skin conditions, meeting both individual needs and aesthetic objectives. Common conditions that are treated with cosmetic lasers are wrinkles, fine lines, age spots, acne scars, vascular lesions, and unwanted hair. A particular type of laser treatment may be necessary for each condition to address its underlying causes and attain the desired improvements in skin tone, texture, and appearance.

When it comes to pigmentation problems like age spots and sun damage, lasers like IPL (Intense Pulsed Light) or Q-switched lasers selectively target melanin in the skin, breaking down excess pigment and promoting even skin tone. Ablative or non-ablative lasers are also effective in treating acne scars because they remodel scar tissue and encourage the formation of new collagen for smoother skin texture. Laser treatments for wrinkles and fine lines typically use fractional lasers, which deliver microscopic laser beams to stimulate collagen production and tighten skin.

Knowing what conditions can be treated with lasers allows people to investigate focused solutions for their skincare issues. Speaking with a certified dermatologist or laser specialist guarantees customized treatment plans that prioritize skin health and safety over results optimization. By utilizing cutting-edge laser technologies, people can improve their overall confidence and well-being and attain clearer, more radiant skin.

HOW SKINCARE LASERS OPERATE

By delivering precise wavelengths and energy levels, lasers can achieve controlled tissue effects without affecting surrounding healthy skin. Laser treatments use concentrated light energy to penetrate the skin's layers and target specific chromophores, such as hemoglobin or melanin, depending on the treatment goal. This targeted approach allows lasers to heat and destroy unwanted cells or stimulate beneficial cellular responses, such as collagen production.

Different laser types and treatment modalities have different mechanisms of action. Ablative lasers, for example, stimulate regeneration and improve texture by removing outer layers of skin; non-ablative lasers, on the other hand, penetrate deeper into the dermis to tighten underlying tissues and promote collagen remodeling without causing surface damage; fractional lasers deliver microscopic treatment zones while sparing surrounding tissue, which speeds up healing and reduces downtime.

Understanding how lasers work in skincare highlights their versatility and precision in addressing a wide range of aesthetic concerns. With cutting-edge laser technologies and creative treatment protocols, efficacy and patient comfort are enhanced.

Contemporary laser systems frequently incorporate cooling mechanisms to protect the skin's surface and optimize treatment outcomes. This integrated approach guarantees that each laser session is not only effective in achieving cosmetic goals but also safe and comfortable for the patient.

SAFETY OBSERVATIONS AND SAFETY MEASURES

A thorough consultation with a qualified provider is recommended before undergoing cosmetic laser treatments to assess candidacy, go over medical history, and set realistic expectations. This initial assessment also helps identify any contraindications or factors that may affect treatment safety and efficacy. Although cosmetic laser treatments are generally safe and effective, it is important to understand potential risks and precautions to minimize adverse effects and optimize outcomes.

Sun exposure should be avoided before and after treatments to minimize the risk of hyperpigmentation and ensure optimal healing. Skin type, sensitivity, and pre-existing medical conditions that may influence treatment outcomes are among the safety considerations. People with darker skin tones or specific medical conditions may require customized laser settings to minimize the risk of pigmentary changes or other complications.

Regular follow-up appointments allow providers to monitor progress, address any concerns, and adjust treatment plans as needed to ensure ongoing satisfaction and safety. Protective eyewear is typically worn during laser sessions to shield the eyes from intense light, and topical anesthetics or skin cooling devices may be used to enhance comfort during treatment. Post-treatment care instructions, such as gentle cleansing, moisturizing, and sun protection, are provided to support skin recovery and maximize results.

CHAPTER THREE
COSMETIC LASER TREATMENT TYPES
LASER ACNE AND ACNE SCAR TREATMENTS

Acne, a common condition caused by clogged pores and bacteria, can leave behind scars that affect skin texture and appearance. Laser treatments target acne by reducing oil production and killing acne-causing bacteria deep within the skin. This process helps prevent future breakouts and promotes clearer skin over time. Laser treatments for acne and acne scars offer effective solutions for those struggling with persistent skin issues.

Different types of lasers are used depending on the severity of the scars and the type of skin: ablative lasers remove thin layers of skin to reveal smoother skin underneath, while non-ablative lasers penetrate deeper layers without damaging the surface, stimulating collagen production. These lasers work by remodeling the skin's surface and improving the appearance of scars by smoothing out uneven texture and reducing discoloration.

A dermatologist evaluates the condition of the patient's skin before prescribing the best type of laser. The skin is prepped with numbing cream to reduce discomfort during the procedure. The laser produces controlled bursts of light that target specific areas of concern. Following the procedure, the patient must protect the skin from the sun and adhere to the dermatologist's recommended skincare routine to maximize results. A few treatments are often enough to produce noticeable results, though many patients report seeing results after just a few sessions.

TECHNIQUES FOR LASER HAIR REMOVAL

To achieve permanent hair reduction in a variety of body areas, laser hair removal is a popular procedure that targets hair follicles, as opposed to traditional methods like shaving or waxing, which only produce temporary results. The process involves shining concentrated light into the hair follicles, which absorbs the light and damages the follicle enough to prevent future growth. It is effective on both large and small areas, including the face, legs, underarms, and bikini line.

Before treatment, the area is shaved and cleaned to prepare for laser application. Patients may experience a slight tingling sensation or mild discomfort during the procedure, which is usually well-tolerated. There are various types of lasers available, each suitable for different skin tones and hair types. The laser's wavelength is adjusted based on skin color and hair thickness to ensure optimal results and minimize the risk of skin damage.

It takes several sessions to effectively target hair follicles in their active growth phase. Maintenance sessions may be necessary on occasion to maintain smooth, hair-free skin. Laser hair removal offers a convenient and effective solution for reducing unwanted hair growth, offering long-lasting results with minimal maintenance. The treated area may appear red and feel sensitive, similar to a mild sunburn. This subsides within a few hours to a few days. Over the following weeks, hair sheds as the damaged follicles release the treated hairs.

AGE-REDUCING LASER PROCEDURES

Laser resurfacing treatments function by targeting the deeper layers of the skin, where collagen and elastin fibers reside, promoting natural regeneration and smoothing out wrinkles. Anti-aging laser treatments use advanced technology to rejuvenate the skin, reducing signs of aging such as wrinkles, fine lines, and uneven skin tone. These treatments also improve skin elasticity and stimulate collagen production, promoting a more youthful appearance.

Non-ablative lasers, like IPL (Intense Pulsed Light) and fractional lasers, penetrate the skin without damaging the outer layer, making them suitable for mild to moderate signs of aging. Fractional lasers, like CO_2 and erbium lasers, are commonly used for anti-aging treatments. These lasers create microscopic wounds in the skin, stimulating collagen production and triggering the skin's healing process for smoother texture, tighter skin, and reducing wrinkles over time.

Before treatment, a dermatologist consultation helps determine the best type of laser and treatment plan based on the patient's skin condition and desired results. During the procedure, the skin is made comfortable by applying a topical anesthetic. The laser is then applied to the targeted areas, producing controlled light pulses that stimulate collagen production and improve skin texture. The post-treatment care involves avoiding sun exposure and adhering to the dermatologist's recommended skincare regimen to maximize results. The procedure may require multiple sessions to achieve the desired results, with noticeable improvements appearing gradually over weeks.

PROCEDURES FOR LASER TATTOO REMOVAL

With minimal scarring, high-intensity light beams from a specialized laser are used to break down tattoo ink particles; depending on the color of the ink, different light wavelengths are used to target each pigment specifically and fragment it into smaller pieces. Laser tattoo removal is a safe and efficient method of getting rid of unwanted tattoos.

To achieve complete removal, several sessions are usually needed, spaced several weeks apart to allow the skin to heal in between treatments. During the procedure, the laser is passed over the tattooed area, delivering rapid pulses of light that penetrate the skin and target the ink. The energy from the laser causes the ink particles to heat up and shatter into tiny fragments, which the body's immune system naturally removes over time, gradually fading the tattoo.

Several factors determine the number of sessions required, such as the size, color, and depth of the tattoo, as well as the patient's skin type and immune response. Topical anesthetic creams can be applied ahead of time to minimize discomfort. Following each session, the treated area may appear red, swollen, or blistered, resembling a mild sunburn that goes away in a few hours to a few days. Adequate aftercare, such as keeping the area clean and shielded from the sun, aids in the healing process and lowers the likelihood of complications.

TREATMENTS FOR VASCULAR LESIONS AND PIGMENTATION

Pigmentation problems like sunspots, melasma, and freckles are caused by an excess of melanin in the skin; vascular lesions, such as spider veins and broken capillaries, are caused by the dilation of blood vessels near the skin's surface. Melanin or hemoglobin (the pigment in blood) is the target of laser treatments for pigmentation and vascular lesions, which improve overall skin tone and texture by targeting skin discoloration and visible blood vessels.

Depending on the particular condition being treated and the type of skin, different types of lasers are used: IPL (Intense Pulsed Light) or Q-switched lasers are used for pigmentation issues; these lasers emit light energy that is absorbed by the skin's melanin, causing it to fragment and fade over time; for vascular lesions. Hemoglobin is the target of lasers, which cause blood vessels to coagulate and become less visible.

Before treatment, a dermatologist assesses the patient's skin condition and determines the best type and settings for the laser. The laser is applied to the targeted area, delivering precise pulses of light to treat pigmented spots or vascular lesions. The procedure is usually well-tolerated, and patients may experience mild discomfort. Following treatment, the skin may appear slightly red or swollen, resembling a mild sunburn, but this usually goes away in a few hours to a few days. Multiple sessions may be necessary to get the best results, with improvements becoming apparent as the skin heals and the pigmentation fades.

CHAPTER FOUR

SELECTING THE APPROPRIATE LASER THERAPY

KNOWING YOUR SKIN TYPE AND IF IT'S GOOD FOR LASERS

Understanding your skin type and how well it responds to various laser types is the first step in selecting the appropriate laser treatment. Skin types vary from extremely fair to dark, and each type responds to laser therapy differently. For example, fair skin is usually more responsive to laser treatments because of the higher contrast between skin and hair color, which makes it easier for lasers to target hair follicles.

On the other hand, darker skin tones necessitate lasers that are specifically made to reduce the risk of pigmentation changes.

Based on color, sensitivity to sun exposure, and tendency to tan or burn, the Fitzpatrick Scale divides skin into six categories:

Type VI is very dark, and Type I is very fair. Based on this scale, laser therapists can determine the best type of laser and settings for each patient; for example, people with Type I to III skin can usually benefit from treatments with Alexandrite or Diode lasers because they efficiently target melanin in hair follicles with little risk to the surrounding skin.

To achieve safe and effective results, it is important to understand your skin type and how it responds to laser therapy. Speaking with a dermatologist or licensed clinician with experience in laser treatments can help you determine which type of laser is best for your skin type and hair color.

This initial consultation will help you customize your treatment plan and make sure the laser you choose will target hair follicles effectively while minimizing side effects on your skin.

PROCESS OF CONSULTATION WITH A CLINICIAN OR DERMATOLOGIST

A crucial first step in selecting the best cosmetic laser treatment is scheduling a consultation with a dermatologist or clinician. In this consultation, your skin type, hair color, medical history, and treatment objectives will be evaluated to identify the best option for laser therapy. The dermatologist will also thoroughly inquire about any medications you take, your skin care regimen, and any prior cosmetic procedures you've had.

The consultation is also an opportunity to address any concerns or questions you may have regarding the procedure, recovery time, and expected results. In addition, a patch test may be performed to evaluate how your skin responds to the laser and to determine the appropriate laser settings for your particular needs.

Overall, the consultation process aims to establish a clear understanding between you and your healthcare provider, ensuring a personalized treatment plan that meets your needs and meets your expectations. The dermatologist or clinician will explain the potential risks and benefits associated with the chosen laser treatment, including possible side effects like redness, swelling, or temporary pigment changes. They will also provide post-treatment care instructions to maximize results and minimize discomfort.

FACTORS AFFECTING THE EFFECTIVENESS OF TREATMENT

Skin type is one of the most important factors that affect how effective cosmetic laser treatments are; darker skin tones require lasers that emit longer wavelengths to prevent damage to the skin's pigment cells. Hair color also has an impact on treatment effectiveness; darker hair absorbs more laser energy than lighter hair colors, which makes it easier to target the hair follicle for removal.

Coarse hair is more responsive to laser treatments than fine hair because of its larger diameter and greater pigment content. Other factors to take into account include the density and thickness of the hair in the treatment area. The number of treatment sessions required for optimal results varies depending on these factors and the individual's response to the laser therapy.

A qualified professional can adjust the laser settings according to the patient's skin type and hair color, ensuring effective treatment while minimizing the risk of complications. Adequate pre-treatment preparation and post-treatment care further enhance the overall effectiveness and safety of the laser therapy, ensuring satisfactory results. The skill and experience of the clinician performing the procedure also impact treatment outcomes.

TAILORING INTERVENTIONS TO INDIVIDUAL REQUIREMENTS

Following a thorough evaluation of the patient's skin type, hair color, and medical history during the initial consultation, the clinician selects the most appropriate laser type and settings to achieve optimal results while ensuring safety and minimal discomfort. Personalized laser treatment planning entails customizing the procedure to address specific concerns and desired outcomes.

To achieve gradual hair reduction and smoother skin, a customized treatment plan may include multiple sessions spaced several weeks apart, to adjust laser parameters such as pulse duration and energy level to target hair follicles effectively without causing damage to surrounding tissues. For example, individuals with sensitive skin may benefit from lasers that offer cooling mechanisms to reduce heat and discomfort during treatment.

Additionally, depending on the patient's response to laser therapy and their specific aesthetic goals, other treatments or complementary therapies might be suggested. These could include topical treatments, skincare regimens, or maintenance sessions to extend the results of laser hair removal. By tailoring treatments to each patient's needs, clinicians can guarantee patient satisfaction and the long-term success of cosmetic laser therapies.

CONTROLLING RESULTS AND EXPECTATIONS

While laser therapy offers effective hair reduction, individual results may vary based on factors such as skin type, hair color, and hair density. During the consultation, the dermatologist or clinician will discuss realistic expectations based on your unique characteristics and treatment goals. Managing expectations and understanding potential results are essential aspects of undergoing cosmetic laser treatments.

It's crucial to understand that laser hair removal usually takes several sessions to produce noticeable hair reduction.

Most patients notice a gradual decrease in hair growth with each session, which eventually results in smoother skin. Results may not be apparent right away following the first treatment session, but they will become more apparent as the sessions go on.

Understanding potential side effects and transient changes, like redness, swelling, or mild discomfort, that may happen after laser treatments and that usually go away in a few hours to a few days is another way to manage expectations. It's also important to keep realistic expectations about how long results will last and whether or not future maintenance sessions will be necessary to guarantee a positive experience with the procedure and satisfactory results.

CHAPTER FIVE

GETTING READY FOR A LASER PROCEDURE

SKINCARE ROUTINE BEFORE TREATMENT

For the best results and the least amount of side effects, prepare your skin before a cosmetic laser treatment. Wash your face well with a mild cleanser to get rid of any debris, oil, or makeup residues. Then, gently exfoliate your skin to make sure that dead skin cells are gone and to allow the laser to penetrate the skin evenly. Avoid using harsh scrubs or exfoliants as this could aggravate your skin before the treatment.

Consider using a hydrating mask or serum containing ingredients like hyaluronic acid to boost your skin's moisture levels and prepare it for the laser session. After cleansing and exfoliating, apply a soothing moisturizer to hydrate and protect your skin. Choose a moisturizer that is gentle and suitable for sensitive skin types to avoid any potential irritation post-treatment.

This last step in the pre-treatment skincare regimen will help guarantee that your skin is in the best possible condition for the laser treatment, promoting effective results and minimizing the risk of adverse reactions.

Sun protection is essential both before and after laser treatment to prevent hyperpigmentation and other complications. Remember to reapply sunscreen throughout the day, especially if you'll be outdoors.

KEEPING OUT OF THE SUN AND TAKING OTHER PRECAUTIONS

If you must be outside in the days before your cosmetic laser treatment, wear protective clothing, and a wide-brimmed hat, and seek shade whenever possible. You should also avoid using tanning beds or self-tanning products that can darken the skin because UV rays can make your skin more sensitive and increase the risk of complications such as burns or hyperpigmentation from the laser.

The sensitivity of your skin to laser treatment can also be influenced by certain medications and skincare products. Please let your healthcare provider know about all the medications you take, including oral and topical creams, to make sure they won't interfere with the procedure; some medications, like retinoids or antibiotics, may need to be stopped temporarily before treatment.

The days before your appointment, keep up a gentle skincare routine. Steer clear of harsh chemicals, strong acids, or abrasive scrubs that might irritate your skin. To get the most out of your cosmetic laser therapy, follow any special instructions given by your healthcare provider regarding pre-treatment preparations.

POSSIBLE ADVERSE REACTIONS AND THEIR HANDLING

Knowing what to anticipate and how to effectively manage any side effects can help you prepare for cosmetic laser therapy.

Common side effects after treatment include mild discomfort, redness, and swelling; these effects are usually transient and go away in a few hours to a few days.

Your healthcare provider may advise using a light moisturizer or topical ointment to keep the skin hydrated and speed up the healing process. To manage redness and swelling, apply a cold compress or ice pack wrapped in a cloth to the treated area. This can help reduce inflammation and soothe the skin. Avoid touching or picking at the treated area to prevent infection and further irritation.

Contact your healthcare provider right away if you experience any concerning symptoms or if side effects worsen over time. They can offer guidance on appropriate treatments or medications to relieve discomfort and promote healing. In rare cases, more severe side effects like blistering, scarring, or changes in skin pigmentation may occur.

MENTAL READINESS FOR THE INTERVENTION PROCEDURE

Cosmetic laser treatment can be mentally prepared for by knowing what to expect from the procedure, controlling expectations, and keeping a positive outlook. You should also educate yourself about the particular type of laser treatment you will receive, including how it works and what kind of results you can realistically expect. This will help to reduce any anxiety or uncertainty you may have about the procedure.

Knowing what to expect during the treatment can help you feel more confident and prepared on the day of your appointment.

Visualize a successful treatment outcome and concentrate on the benefits of undergoing laser therapy, such as improved skin texture, and reduced wrinkles, or acne scars. If you have any questions or concerns, don't hesitate to discuss them with your healthcare provider.

To ensure that your body and mind are in optimal condition for treatment, arrive at your appointment well-rested and hydrated.

You can approach the cosmetic laser therapy process with a positive attitude and improve the overall experience by practicing relaxation techniques like deep breathing or meditation to reduce stress and promote a calm state of mind before and during the procedure.

THINGS TO PACK AND KNOW BEFORE TREATMENT DAY

Wear comfortable clothing that allows easy access to the treatment area and refrain from applying makeup or skincare products on the treated area, unless your healthcare provider instructs you to do so. These are important preparations for your cosmetic laser treatment.

Bring any prescription drugs or skincare products your doctor has prescribed for use right after the treatment, such as calming lotions, ointments, or sunscreen; also, pack a cap or scarf to shield your skin from the sun on the walk home.

Your laser treatment session will take place in a clinic or healthcare facility; the length of time will depend on the size of the treatment area and the type of laser being used. Before starting, your healthcare provider will go over each step of the procedure and answer any last-minute questions or concerns you may have.

Following the procedure, your doctor will give you post-care instructions that you should carefully follow to encourage healing and get the most out of your cosmetic laser therapy session. These instructions will cover how to take care of your skin, how to handle any side effects, and when to make follow-up appointments.

CHAPTER SIX

COURSE OF THE LASER TREATMENT

DETAILED PROCESS OF AN ORDINARY LASER SESSION

Your clinician will usually cleanse your skin to remove debris, oils, and makeup that could interfere with the effectiveness of the laser before starting a laser treatment session. If necessary, they may also apply a numbing cream, especially for sensitive areas or if you have a low pain threshold. After your skin is prepared, you will be given protective eyewear to shield your eyes from the laser's light.

The treatment involves the use of a handheld laser device by the clinician to apply concentrated beams of light to specific areas of your skin, with the intensity and duration of each application carefully monitored. The laser may cause a sensation similar to that of a rubber band snapping against your skin, or it may cause a warm, prickling sensation as it targets hair follicles or skin imperfections.

After a few minutes to an hour, depending on the type of laser used and the treatment area, the clinician will apply a cooling gel or use a cooling device to minimize discomfort and soothe the treated area. After the session, they will provide post-treatment care instructions, which usually include avoiding sun exposure and applying soothing creams or moisturizers to help with recovery.

FEELINGS OF UNCOMFORT DURING MEDICAL INTERVENTION

As the laser pulses target the skin during a laser treatment session, you may experience a variety of sensations, some mild to moderate and comparable to tiny pinpricks or the feeling of a rubber band snapping against the skin. These sensations can vary depending on the type of laser used and the sensitivity of the treatment area.

Some discomfort is possible for more sensitive areas or people with lower pain thresholds, especially for hair removal or treatments aimed at deeper skin layers. Physicians typically offer options to minimize discomfort, such as numbing cream applications before the procedure. During the procedure, cooling devices or chilled air may be used to relieve any heat or discomfort caused by the laser.

Any discomfort you experience during the session should be discussed openly with your clinician so they can make any necessary adjustments to the settings or techniques. Most people resume their daily activities immediately following treatment, and any discomfort usually goes away quite quickly.

SAFETY PROCEDURES THAT PRACTITIONERS ADHERE TO

Strict adherence to established safety protocols by qualified professionals is necessary to ensure your safety during laser treatments. Before the procedure, your clinician will perform a comprehensive evaluation of your skin type, medical history, and potential contraindications for laser therapy. This assessment aids in determining the best type of laser and settings for your skin type and treatment objectives.

Throughout the procedure, the clinician will monitor your comfort level and wear protective eyewear to shield your eyes from the light of the laser. They will also make sure you have the proper eye protection to protect your eyes from the laser's light.

Follow-up appointments may be arranged to monitor your skin's response to treatment and make any required adjustments to treatment plans. Following treatment, clinicians provide comprehensive instructions for aftercare, including sun protection and skincare routines to promote healing and minimize any risk of adverse effects like hyperpigmentation or skin irritation.

EFFECTS AND CHANGES SEEN IN REAL-TIME

Some people report a sensation of warmth or tingling, which is normal and part of the skin's natural response to laser energy.

After a laser treatment session, you may notice temporary effects like mild redness or swelling around the treated area. These effects usually go away within a few hours to a day, depending on the intensity of the treatment and your skin's sensitivity.

As the targeted imperfections, like hair follicles or pigmented lesions, start to fade or diminish, you can anticipate gradual improvements in the appearance of your skin over the next few days and weeks. The exact results will depend on the type of treatment you receive and your unique skin type; best results often require several sessions spaced several weeks apart.

Maintaining regular communication with your clinician ensures that any concerns or questions about the observed effects can be addressed promptly. Post-treatment care instructions, which may include avoiding sun exposure, using gentle skincare products, and staying hydrated to support your skin's healing process, are crucial for optimizing results and minimizing potential side effects.

SPEAKING WITH YOUR PHYSICIAN THROUGHOUT THE TREATMENT

To ensure your comfort, safety, and the best possible results from your laser treatment, you must communicate effectively with your clinician. Before the laser treatment session starts, your clinician will go over each step of the process with you and welcome any questions or concerns you may have. This helps build trust and clarity about what to expect during the treatment.

Feel free to share any sensations or discomfort you have during the session. Your clinician can help you relax during the procedure by offering techniques to divert your attention or by adjusting settings or techniques to enhance your comfort and address any unexpected reactions.

Your clinician is there to ensure your safety and satisfaction throughout the session; if you have any questions at all about the treatment or its effects, please ask.

CHAPTER SEVEN
RECUPERATION AND AFTERCARE
AFTER-TREATMENT SKINCARE SCHEDULE

Establishing a dedicated post-treatment skincare routine is essential to maximizing results and promoting healing following cosmetic laser therapy. Following the procedure, your skin will be sensitive and may experience mild swelling or redness.

It is important to adhere to the specific instructions given by your skincare professional or dermatologist. Generally, this entails gently cleansing the treatment area with a mild, non-abrasive cleanser to remove any residue or impurities.

After cleansing, use the calming serum or moisturizer that your skincare professional has recommended. These products help to restore moisture and support the skin's natural barrier function, which may be temporarily compromised after laser therapy. You should also use a broad-spectrum sunscreen with an

SPF of 30 or higher every day, even when you're indoors, to shield your skin from UV rays while it heals.

If you notice any discomfort or strange symptoms, get in touch with your skincare provider right away so they can provide you with advice. As your skin heals over the next few days, keep moisturizing and steer clear of harsh skincare products or exfoliants that might irritate the treated area. By following a regular post-treatment skincare routine, you can maximize the results of your cosmetic laser therapy and preserve healthy, glowing skin.

HANDLING TRANSIENT SIDE EFFECTS LIKE SWELLING OR REDNESS

Depending on the type and intensity of the treatment, temporary side effects like redness or swelling are common following cosmetic laser therapy. Right after the procedure, your skin may appear red or slightly irritated, like a mild sunburn.

This is a normal reaction as the laser energy targets specific skin concerns, like pigmentation or fine lines.

Avoid applying ice directly to the skin to prevent frostbite or further irritation. Instead, use cold compresses or ice packs wrapped in a clean cloth on the affected area. This helps to constrict blood vessels and reduce inflammation, providing immediate relief from redness and swelling. You can also use gentle skincare products designed for sensitive skin to soothe and hydrate the affected area.

Continue to observe your skin's reaction over the next few days, and stay away from activities that might aggravate redness or swelling, like strenuous exercise or exposure to high temperatures. See your skincare provider for specific recommendations if discomfort continues or gets worse. With the right care and attention, transient side effects can go away quickly, letting you take full advantage of cosmetic laser therapy.

REFRAINING FROM ACTIVITIES THAT MAY AFFECT REHAB

In the post-cosmetic laser therapy recovery period, it is imperative to avoid certain activities that may impede healing or jeopardize the results of the procedure. Immediately following the procedure, avoid vigorous exercise, hot showers, or direct sunlight as these can exacerbate skin sensitivity and lengthen the recovery period. Instead, choose gentle activities and protect the treated area from aggressors in the environment.

It is also advised that you abstain from smoking and alcohol consumption, as these behaviors can impede circulation and postpone the healing process of the skin. Additionally, you should exercise caution when applying skincare products or cosmetics on the treated area, choosing gentle formulations devoid of harsh chemicals or fragrances. By following these recommendations, you can promote the healing process that occurs naturally and reduce the likelihood of complications following cosmetic laser therapy.

Prioritizing careful post-procedural care can help you achieve smoother, healthier-looking skin in the long run. If you have any questions or concerns about specific activities to avoid during recovery, speak with your skincare provider for personalized advice based on your skin type, treatment goals, and general health.

APPOINTMENTS FOR FOLLOW-UP AND THEIR SIGNIFICANCE

After cosmetic laser therapy, making and keeping follow-up appointments is crucial to tracking how your skin responds to treatment and achieving the best possible outcomes. Usually, follow-up visits are scheduled a few weeks later to evaluate healing progress, address any concerns, and adjust your skincare routine if needed. Your dermatologist or skincare specialist can monitor improvements in skin tone, texture, and overall appearance during these appointments.

Follow-up appointments offer an opportunity to discuss long-term skincare goals and develop a personalized maintenance plan tailored to your skin's needs. Your provider may perform additional assessments, such as skin analysis or imaging, to evaluate treatment outcomes and determine if further sessions are needed. They may also recommend complementary skincare treatments or products to enhance and maintain your results.

To maintain healthy, radiant skin over time and maximize the benefits of cosmetic laser therapy, you must prioritize regular follow-up appointments. By doing this, you can proactively manage your skincare journey and ensure continued progress toward achieving your desired aesthetic goals. If you experience any unexpected changes or concerns between appointments, don't hesitate to contact your skin care provider for guidance.

TIPS FOR LONG-TERM SKINCARE MAINTENANCE

Developing a thorough, long-term skincare maintenance regimen following cosmetic laser therapy is essential to maintaining your results and fostering skin health. Include sunscreen, moisturizers, and mild cleansers in your daily routine to guard against environmental damage and keep your skin hydrated. Look for products that are packed with vitamins, antioxidants, and hydrating ingredients to revitalize and nourish your skin.

To augment the benefits of laser therapy by accelerating cellular turnover and collagen production, periodic treatments like chemical peels, microdermabrasion, and facials can be incorporated in addition to daily skincare regimens to address specific concerns and improve skin texture. Speak with your skincare provider to receive customized recommendations based on your skin type, concerns, and past treatment history.

Maintaining a consistent skincare routine and forming healthy habits can help you prolong the benefits of cosmetic laser therapy and enjoy youthful, radiant skin for years to come. Other healthy lifestyle priorities include avoiding smoking, excessive alcohol consumption, and prolonged sun exposure, which can accelerate skin aging and diminish treatment results. Finally, prioritize overall skin health from within by adopting a balanced diet, regular exercise, and adequate hydration.

CHAPTER EIGHT

TYPICAL LASER THERAPY CONCERNS

LASER TREATMENT SAFETY FOR VARIOUS SKIN TONES

Since darker skin tones are more susceptible to pigmentation changes and burns from laser treatments because of higher melanin levels, laser therapy has become popular in the skincare industry due to its accuracy and effectiveness in treating a variety of conditions.

That being said, advances in laser technology, such as longer wavelengths and cooling mechanisms, have greatly improved safety profiles for all skin types.

For each skin tone and condition, a qualified dermatologist or laser specialist should be consulted to determine the best laser type and settings. This customized approach improves treatment safety and efficacy, ensuring minimal risk of adverse effects while achieving desired skincare results.

By prioritizing safety through appropriate laser selection and expert guidance, individuals can confidently pursue laser therapy for a variety of skin concerns, knowing they are minimizing risks and maximizing the benefits of advanced skincare technology. Having a thorough understanding of the nuances of laser safety for different skin tones empowers individuals to make informed decisions about their skincare treatments.

THE DANGERS OF LASER THERAPY AND HOW TO REDUCE THEM

Although laser therapy is a useful tool for treating skin care issues, it carries some risks as well. It is important to know what these risks are and how to reduce them to ensure safe and effective treatment outcomes. Common risks include mild pain or stinging sensations that may occur during treatment; these can usually be managed with topical anesthetics or cooling techniques applied both before and during the procedure.

To minimize these risks, choosing a qualified and experienced practitioner is essential. They should conduct a thorough assessment of skin type, medical history, and treatment goals before recommending a suitable laser type and setting.

Additionally, adhering to pre-treatment instructions, such as avoiding sun exposure and certain skincare products, helps prepare the skin and reduce potential adverse reactions. Serious risks include burns, blisters, or changes in skin pigmentation, especially for those with darker skin tones or improper laser settings.

Consistent follow-up appointments enable practitioners to assess skin response and modify treatment parameters as needed, guaranteeing safety during the whole laser therapy procedure. Patients can feel comfortable undergoing laser treatments if they take proactive measures to mitigate risks and follow professional advice.

EVALUATING LASER THERAPY IN COMPARISON TO OTHER SKINCARE PROCEDURES

Among skincare treatments, laser therapy stands out for its accuracy, adaptability, and capacity to effectively target specific skin concerns.

Unlike topical creams or oral medications, lasers can target specific areas of the skin without affecting surrounding tissue, making this targeted approach especially useful for treating conditions like wrinkles, acne scars, and unwanted hair growth, where other treatments may yield less targeted results.

For example, laser skin resurfacing can produce results comparable to chemical peels or microdermabrasion, but with less discomfort and downtime; laser hair removal, on the other hand, offers long-lasting results compared to temporary methods like shaving or waxing, making it an economical and effective choice for hair reduction.

When compared to surgical procedures, laser therapy typically offers faster recovery times and fewer complications.

However, every treatment modality has pros and cons that should be taken into account based on the individual's skin type, concerns, and desired results. Speaking with a skincare specialist can help identify the best course of action based on these factors, guaranteeing maximum satisfaction and results. By knowing how laser therapy differs from other skincare treatments, people can make well-informed decisions to safely and effectively achieve their desired skin goals.

DISPELLING MYTHS AND FALSE BELIEFS REGARDING LASER TREATMENTS

Most people can resume their daily activities immediately after treatment, with only mild redness or swelling that usually subsides within a few hours to days. One common myth about laser treatments is that they are painful and require extended downtime.

While some discomfort during treatment is possible, advancements in laser technology, such as integrated cooling systems, minimize discomfort and reduce recovery times significantly.

An additional misconception regarding laser safety, especially for darker skin tones, is that older laser technologies were more likely to cause pigmentation changes in darker skin; however, more recent lasers with longer wavelengths and adjustable settings are safer and more effective for all skin types. Speaking with a qualified dermatologist or laser specialist ensures accurate assessment and customized treatment plans that minimize any possible risks.

Concerns about cost are also common; some people think that laser treatments are too expensive. Although the initial outlay may seem high, particularly for larger treatment areas or multiple sessions, the long-term advantages of lower skincare products and maintenance costs usually exceed the outlay. To make treatments more affordable, some clinics also offer financing options or package deals.

Debunking these myths with factual information and professional advice allows people to think of laser therapy as a practical solution for their skincare issues. Knowing the truth about laser treatments—such as their safety, discomfort, affordability, and effectiveness for various skin types—allows people to pursue treatments with confidence that meet their objectives and expectations.

COMPREHENDING INSURANCE COVERAGE AND FINANCIAL INVESTMENT

The cost of laser treatments can vary greatly depending on factors like the type of laser used, the size of the treatment area, and the number of sessions required. Initial consultations with skincare specialists typically include cost breakdowns and options for payment plans or package deals to accommodate individual budgets.

Insurance coverage for laser therapy varies and is frequently based on the particular condition being treated. Some medical conditions treated with lasers, like vascular lesions or precancerous skin growths, may qualify for partial coverage depending on insurance policies and medical necessity. Cosmetic procedures, like laser hair removal or skin rejuvenation, are typically not covered by insurance because they are considered elective treatments.

Having a clear understanding of these financial factors enables patients to make appropriate plans and look into ways to reduce the cost of laser therapy. For example, some clinics provide financing options or discounts for bundled treatments, which facilitates budgeting for multiple sessions. Keeping lines of communication open with healthcare providers regarding insurance coverage and payment options also helps prevent unanticipated expenses.

Understanding the financial landscape of laser therapy improves the planning process and supports a positive treatment experience for patients seeking medical treatments or cosmetic improvements.

CHAPTER NINE

FREQUENTLY ASKED QUESTIONS ON COSMETIC LASER TREATMENT

HOW MANY APPOINTMENTS ARE USUALLY REQUIRED?

Several weeks separate each session to give the skin enough time to heal and regenerate. The number of sessions needed for cosmetic laser therapy depends on the particular condition being treated and the type of laser used. For example, superficial skin issues like fine lines, minor scars, or uneven pigmentation may only require a few sessions, usually three to six. More severe skin issues like deep scars, significant pigmentation issues, or vascular lesions may require a longer treatment plan, often involving eight or more sessions.

A dermatologist or laser specialist consultation is essential to determine the right number of sessions. They will evaluate the patient's skin type, assess the condition of the skin, and recommend a customized treatment plan. The number of sessions will depend on several factors, including the desired outcome, the type of laser used, and the patient's skin response to treatment. Follow-up visits are necessary to track progress and make necessary adjustments to the treatment plan.

Maintaining regularity and following the recommended treatment plan is essential for the best outcomes. Patients should have reasonable expectations and realize that improvements take time. Following the initial series of treatments, some patients may benefit from sporadic maintenance sessions to maintain and improve the results, usually once or twice a year.

IS IT POSSIBLE TO COMBINE LASER TREATMENTS WITH OTHER PROCEDURES?

Combining laser treatments with other cosmetic procedures can improve overall results and address multiple concerns at the same time. For example, laser therapy can be used to improve skin texture, tone, and clarity in conjunction with chemical peels, microdermabrasion, or microneedling; these complementary treatments help exfoliate the skin, which makes it easier for the laser to penetrate deeper and perform more effectively.

Combining laser therapy with injectables like Botox or dermal fillers can yield a more comprehensive rejuvenation by addressing both surface imperfections and deeper structural concerns. Laser therapy targets issues like pigmentation and fine lines, while Botox relaxes facial muscles to reduce wrinkles, and fillers restore volume and contour to the face.

To ensure that each procedure complements the other and results in smoother, more youthful-looking skin, it is crucial to coordinate with a skilled practitioner who can create a cohesive treatment plan tailored to individual needs. They will schedule treatments in a way that maximizes benefits while minimizing downtime and potential side effects.

HOW IS PAIN HANDLED DURING LASER THERAPY? IS LASER THERAPY PAINFUL?

Cosmetic laser therapy is generally well tolerated, though the degree of discomfort varies based on the type of laser used and the patient's pain threshold. Many patients describe the sensation as mild snapping or tingling, akin to the snap of a rubber band against the skin; areas like the face, which have more nerve endings and thinner skin than other parts of the body, maybe more sensitive than other areas.

To minimize discomfort and protect the skin, some advanced laser systems also incorporate cooling devices or use cold air. Following treatment, patients may experience some redness, swelling, or a sunburn-like sensation, but these symptoms usually go away in a few days. Practitioners usually manage discomfort by applying a topical anesthetic cream to the treatment area before the procedure.

Following post-care instructions, such as applying soothing creams or using ice packs, can also help alleviate any lingering discomfort and promote faster healing. Pain management is an essential component of the treatment plan, and patients should communicate openly with their practitioner about their pain levels and any concerns. This allows the practitioner to adjust the treatment settings or recommend additional pain relief measures if necessary.

WHAT DISTINGUISHES THE DIFFERENT LASER TECHNOLOGIES?

Ablative lasers, like CO_2 and Erbium lasers, work by removing the outer layers of the skin to promote collagen production and reveal smoother, younger-looking skin underneath. These lasers are highly effective for treating deep wrinkles, significant sun damage, and scars but usually require a longer recovery period. Different types of laser technologies are designed to target specific skin concerns, so choosing the appropriate laser for the desired outcome is crucial.

Compared to ablative lasers, fractional lasers usually have less downtime but may require more sessions to achieve desired results. Fractional lasers, which can be ablative or non-ablative, create micro-injuries in the skin to stimulate natural healing processes, effectively treating fine lines, texture irregularities, and pigmentation.

And Alexandrite lasers penetrate deeper into the skin without damaging the surface. They are ideal for treating issues such as pigmentation, spider veins, and hair removal.

A skilled laser specialist can help determine which laser is best for a given patient's needs by offering advice on expected outcomes, potential side effects, and the overall treatment plan. Each laser technology has its advantages and disadvantages, and the choice is based on the patient's skin type, the specific condition being treated, and the desired results.

HOW MUCH TIME DO LASER TREATMENT RESULTS LAST?

In general, results from laser treatments can last anywhere from several months to a few years. For example, treatments targeting pigmentation or vascular lesions can provide long-lasting results, especially if the patient follows a proper skincare regimen and avoids excessive sun exposure. The longevity of laser treatment results varies based on several factors, including the type of laser used, the condition being treated, and the individual's skin type and lifestyle.

To maximize and prolong the benefits of laser therapy, patients are often advised to follow a customized skincare regimen that includes moisturizers, sunscreen, and possibly topical treatments. Periodic maintenance sessions, typically recommended once or twice a year, can help refresh the skin and maintain the improvements achieved from the initial series of treatments. Maintenance is essential to maintaining the results.

Lifestyle decisions also have a big influence on how long results last. People can prolong the benefits of laser treatments by not smoking, eating a healthy diet, and spending as little time in the sun as possible. They can also enjoy the long-term benefits of their treatments by visiting a dermatologist or laser specialist regularly, which guarantees that any new skin issues are promptly addressed and the skin stays in good condition.

CHAPTER TEN

FUTURE DIRECTIONS FOR COSMETIC LASER TREATMENT

ADVANCEMENTS IN LASER TECHNOLOGY AND THERAPY METHODS

Innovations in laser technology have led to the development of devices that can target specific skin concerns with greater precision and minimal downtime. For example, fractional lasers now allow practitioners to treat small zones of skin while leaving surrounding tissue intact, promoting faster healing and reducing the risk of side effects.

Additionally, the evolution towards more compact and versatile laser devices has expanded the range of conditions that can be effectively addressed, from pigmentation issues to acne scars and wrinkles. In the field of cosmetic laser therapy, ongoing technological advancements have revolutionized treatment techniques, making procedures safer, more effective, and more accessible.

In addition, the incorporation of various wavelengths and modalities into laser systems has increased their adaptability and effectiveness. Combination therapies, for instance, that combine various laser types or other modalities, such as radiofrequency, have gained popularity and provide all-encompassing solutions for patients with a variety of cosmetic concerns. These advancements not only enhance treatment outcomes but also more effectively address individual skin types and conditions. As technology advances, even more advanced laser platforms may be developed in the future, which may further minimize discomfort, shorten treatment times, and increase the range of conditions that can be treated in cosmetic dermatology.

NEW DEVELOPMENTS IN NON-INVASIVE COSMETIC SURGERY

Technology breakthroughs that enable effective results without invasive incisions have led to a surge in the popularity of non-invasive cosmetic procedures because of their minimal downtime and lower risk than traditional surgical options. Procedures like intense pulsed light (IPL) therapy, laser skin resurfacing, and ultrasound-based treatments like HIFU (High-Intensity Focused Ultrasound) have gained popularity because of their ability to rejuvenate skin, tighten tissues, and improve overall skin texture.

Furthermore, due to advancements in technology such as laser lipolysis and cryolipolysis (fat freezing), demand for non-invasive body contouring treatments has surged. These procedures allow patients to achieve targeted fat reduction and body sculpting without surgery, making them attractive to those seeking aesthetic enhancements with short recovery times. As a result, the future of non-invasive cosmetic procedures appears bright, with advancements in patient comfort, efficacy, and customization of treatment plans based on individual needs and goals expected.

COMBINING ROBOTICS AND AI FOR LASER TREATMENTS

AI algorithms can analyze patient data, skin characteristics, and treatment histories to recommend customized laser settings for optimal results. This capability not only improves treatment accuracy but also lowers the margin for human error, ensuring consistent and reliable outcomes across different patients and skin types. Artificial intelligence (AI) and robotics are increasingly being integrated into cosmetic laser treatments to enhance precision, optimize treatment outcomes, and personalize patient care.

Further, robotics is essential to laser procedures because it can automate repetitive tasks and perform precise maneuvers that are not possible for human hands to accomplish. Robotic-assisted lasers can deliver treatments with unparalleled accuracy, minimizing tissue damage and maximizing therapeutic benefits. The combination of robotics and artificial intelligence in cosmetic laser therapy not only raises the bar for care but also creates opportunities for future treatment modalities and applications. As these technologies advance, their integration is poised to change the face of cosmetic dermatology by providing patients with safer, more effective, and customized treatment experiences.

USING DIGITAL TOOLS TO EMPOWER AND EDUCATE PATIENTS

Websites, mobile apps, and virtual reality simulations now give patients insights into treatment options, expected outcomes, and potential risks, empowering them to make informed decisions about their cosmetic goals.

Additionally, online communities and social media platforms allow patients to share their treatment experiences, connect with others undergoing similar procedures, and seek advice from healthcare professionals. These digital tools have completely changed the way cosmetic laser therapy patients are educated and empowered.

Moreover, digital platforms enable telemedicine and remote consultations, enabling patients to see dermatologists and cosmetic surgeons from the comfort of their homes. This accessibility expands access to specialized care and improves convenience, especially for patients who live in remote areas or have limited mobility. By utilizing digital tools, healthcare providers can improve treatment adherence, foster a supportive environment where patients feel empowered throughout their cosmetic journey, and improve patient satisfaction. In the future, the combination of virtual reality and artificial intelligence will revolutionize patient education by providing immersive experiences that imitate treatment outcomes and lead patients through personalized treatment plans.

ETHICS AND ENVIRONMENTAL ASPECTS OF LASER THERAPY

In the field of cosmetic laser therapy, the trend toward sustainability and ethical practices has also affected clinicians and manufacturers, leading them to prioritize environmentally friendly solutions and ethical considerations in treatment protocols. Sustainable practices, like cutting down on energy consumption and waste in the manufacturing and operation of laser devices, are becoming more and more significant. Additionally, there is an increasing focus on the ethical sourcing of materials used in laser treatments, making sure that products are sourced responsibly and do not contribute to environmental degradation or harm.

In addition, ethical considerations also pertain to patient care and safety, with healthcare providers placing a strong emphasis on openness, informed consent, and ethical treatment practices. These practices encompass upholding professional standards of care throughout the treatment process, respecting patient autonomy, preserving confidentiality, and promoting sustainability. As consumer awareness of environmental and ethical issues grows, the cosmetic dermatology community is working together to adopt practices that prioritize patient well-being, minimize ecological footprint, and promote sustainability. By adhering to these principles, the future of cosmetic laser therapy aims to not only provide superior aesthetic results but also uphold ethical standards and environmental stewardship in healthcare delivery.